This book was compiled by Daniel Melehi
with the A.I assistance of Inventabot

<u>Dedication</u>

I hope this helps all of my wonderful readers achieve all their goals in their business. And I would like to thank my wonderful wife for all of her continued support in all my ventures.

©Daniel Melehi

May 7 2023

Contents

Chapter 1: Understanding Tuberous Sclerosis Complex

Tuberous Sclerosis Complex (TSC) is a genetic disorder that affects various parts of the body, including the brain, heart, kidneys, lungs, and skin. TSC is caused by mutations in the TSC1 or TSC2 gene and affects 1 in 6,000-10,000 individuals worldwide.

SUBCHAPTER 1.1: WHAT IS TUBEROUS SCLEROSIS COMPLEX?

TSC causes non-cancerous tumors to grow in various organs and parts of the body. These tumors can cause a wide range of symptoms that vary from person to person. The severity of TSC can also vary widely, even among individuals with the same genetic mutation.

SUBCHAPTER 1.2: SIGNS AND SYMPTOMS

The signs and symptoms of TSC can appear at any age, and they can vary depending on the type and location of the tumors. Some common symptoms include seizures, cognitive impairment, behavioral issues, skin abnormalities, and kidney problems. Individuals with TSC may also have a higher risk of developing certain types of cancer.

SUBCHAPTER 1.3: CAUSES AND RISK FACTORS

TSC is caused by mutations in the TSC1 or TSC2 gene, which are responsible for producing proteins that regulate cell growth and division. These mutations can be inherited from one or both parents or can occur spontaneously during early development. Risk factors for TSC include having a family history of the disorder or having a parent with TSC. However, in many cases, TSC occurs spontaneously without any family history. In conclusion, Tuberous Sclerosis Complex is a genetic disorder that can cause a variety of symptoms and affect multiple parts of the body. It is caused by mutations in the TSC1 or TSC2 gene and can be inherited or occur spontaneously. In the next chapter, we will explore the different methods of diagnosing TSC.

SUBCHAPTER 1.1: WHAT IS TUBEROUS SCLEROSIS COMPLEX?

Tuberous sclerosis complex (TSC) is a rare genetic disorder that affects multiple organs in the body, including the brain, skin, kidneys, heart, lungs, and eyes. It is caused by mutations in the TSC1 and TSC2 genes, which are responsible for regulating cell growth and division. The mutations in the TSC genes can result in the formation of benign tumors, or growths, in the affected organs. These tumors can cause a variety of symptoms, ranging from mild to severe, depending on their size and location. TSC can affect both children and adults, and it is estimated to occur in about 1 in 6,000 live births. Although there is no cure for TSC, there are treatments available to manage the symptoms and improve the quality of life for those affected by the condition. Common symptoms of TSC include seizures, intellectual disability, developmental delays, behavioral problems, skin abnormalities, and kidney disease. Because TSC affects multiple organs, the symptoms and severity can vary widely from person to person. If you or a loved one has been diagnosed with TSC, it's important to work closely with a medical team that specializes in the condition. This may include a neurologist, dermatologist, urologist, and other specialists as needed to manage the various symptoms and complications associated with TSC. In the next subchapter, we will delve deeper into the signs and symptoms of TSC.

SUBCHAPTER 1.2: SIGNS AND SYMPTOMS

Tuberous Sclerosis Complex (TSC) is a genetic disease that can affect different parts of the body. It is important to recognize the signs and symptoms of TSC early on, so that it can be diagnosed and treated appropriately. One of the hallmark symptoms of TSC is the presence of benign tumors called hamartomas. These tumors can grow in different organs such as the brain, heart, kidneys, and skin. In the brain, these tumors can cause seizures, developmental delays, and intellectual disability. In the heart, they can cause arrhythmias and heart failure. In the kidneys, they can lead to kidney disease and high blood pressure. In the skin, they can cause discolored patches and bumps or acne-like lesions. Other signs and symptoms of TSC that may alert doctors to a potential diagnosis include: - White spots on the skin called hypomelanotic macules - Facial angiofibromas (small, reddish bumps on the face) - Shagreen patches (thick, leathery areas of skin) - Multiple dental pits - Retinal lesions It is important to note that not all individuals with TSC will have all of these symptoms, and some may have only mild or no symptoms at all. However, if these symptoms are observed, it is crucial to consult with a doctor for proper evaluation. In addition to the physical symptoms, TSC can also have an impact on an individual's cognitive and behavioral development. Some individuals with TSC may experience autism spectrum disorder, attention deficit hyperactivity disorder (ADHD), anxiety, and depression. These conditions can be managed with proper treatment and therapy. Overall, recognizing the signs and symptoms of TSC is essential for early diagnosis and treatment. It is important to work closely with a healthcare professional to manage the condition and improve outcomes for those affected by TSC.

SUBCHAPTER 1.3: CAUSES AND RISK FACTORS

Tuberous Sclerosis Complex (TSC) is a genetic disorder and is caused by mutations of the TSC1 and TSC2 genes. These genes are responsible for regulating cell growth and differentiation. Mutations of these genes lead to the formation of benign tumors, which can develop in various organs of the body, including the brain, heart, kidneys, lungs, and skin. TSC is an autosomal dominant genetic disorder, which means that a person can inherit it from one parent who has the mutated gene. However, in most cases, TSC occurs sporadically, which means that the mutation arises spontaneously and is not inherited from either parent. The severity of TSC and the symptoms that the affected person experiences can vary widely even within the same family. This variability is due to a phenomenon called "genetic mosaicism," in which cells in different parts of the body have different mutations of the TSC1 and TSC2 genes. Some people with TSC may never develop symptoms, while others may experience severe symptoms that significantly impact their quality of life. The reason for this variability is still not well understood and is an active area of research. In addition to genetic mutations, certain factors may increase the risk of developing TSC. For example, a family history of the disorder increases the risk of inheriting the mutated gene. Additionally, advanced parental age and certain medical conditions, such as epilepsy and mental retardation, may increase the risk of TSC. It is important to note that TSC is a rare disorder, and not all individuals with risk factors will develop the condition. Nevertheless, for those individuals with risk factors, it is essential to be aware of the signs and symptoms of the disorder and seek medical attention if any symptoms arise. In the next chapter, we will look at the different ways in which TSC can be diagnosed, which is essential for early intervention and effective management of the disorder.

Chapter 2: Diagnosing Tuberous Sclerosis Complex

Tuberous Sclerosis Complex (TSC) is a genetic disorder that affects the growth of benign tumors in various organs of the body, including the brain, heart, kidneys, and lungs. It is often diagnosed through clinical evaluations and a variety of medical tests.

SUBCHAPTER 2.1: DIAGNOSIS IN INFANCY

Diagnosis of TSC in infancy may be based on visible symptoms, such as the presence of seizures or a rash. Doctors may also monitor the growth and development of children who have a family history of TSC or who are at risk for the disorder due to mutations in certain genes. Medical tests may also be conducted to confirm a diagnosis of TSC. Magnetic resonance imaging (MRI), computerized tomography (CT) scans, and electroencephalograms (EEGs) can help identify the presence of tumors, brain abnormalities, and seizures.

SUBCHAPTER 2.2: DIAGNOSIS IN CHILDHOOD

As children with TSC grow and develop, additional symptoms may emerge, such as behavioral and learning difficulties. Diagnosis may be made based on observations of these symptoms, as well as additional medical tests, such as echocardiograms to check for cardiac tumors and urine tests to check for kidney problems. Children with TSC may also undergo eye exams to check for retinal hamartomas, which are benign tumors that can affect vision.

SUBCHAPTER 2.3: DIAGNOSIS IN ADULTHOOD

While TSC is often diagnosed in childhood, some individuals may not receive a diagnosis until later in life. This may occur if they have few or no visible symptoms, or if their symptoms are mistaken for other conditions. Diagnosis in adulthood may involve medical tests, such as MRIs and CT scans, as well as evaluations of symptoms, such as seizures and learning difficulties. Genetic testing may also be conducted to identify mutations that are known to cause TSC and to determine the likelihood of passing the disorder on to offspring. Diagnosing TSC can be a complex process, and individuals who suspect that they or their children may have the disorder should seek out medical professionals with experience in this area. A proper diagnosis can open the door to a range of treatment options and support services that can help individuals with TSC to manage their symptoms and optimize their quality of life.

CHAPTER 2: DIAGNOSING TUBEROUS SCLEROSIS COMPLEX

Subchapter 2.1: Diagnosis in Infancy

Tuberous Sclerosis Complex (TSC) is usually diagnosed in infancy due to the presence of several signs and symptoms. In some cases, it may even be detected before birth through ultrasound. When a child is born with TSC, they may have white patches or bumps on the skin, known as hypomelanotic macules or angiofibromas. They may also have seizures or developmental delays, which can be indicative of TSC. In some cases, TSC may be diagnosed after a seizure occurs and the child undergoes imaging tests such as an MRI or CT scan. These tests can detect the presence of brain tumors, known as tubers, which are a common symptom of TSC. It's important for parents to be vigilant for any signs or symptoms of TSC in their child, especially if there is a family history of the disorder. If you suspect your child may have TSC, it's important to consult with a medical professional as soon as possible. Diagnosing TSC in infancy can be a challenging process, but with early detection and appropriate treatment, children with TSC can lead fulfilling lives. In the next subchapter, we will discuss diagnosis in childhood.

CHAPTER 2: DIAGNOSING TUBEROUS SCLEROSIS COMPLEX

Subchapter 2.2: Diagnosis in Childhood

Diagnosing Tuberous Sclerosis Complex (TSC) in childhood can be challenging due to the wide range of symptoms that can manifest during this period. Children with

TSC may display a variety of symptoms such as seizures, developmental delay, behavioral impairment, and skin abnormalities. Identifying these symptoms early is crucial to provide effective treatment and support. Doctors typically look for the presence of specific TSC features including:

Skin findings

One of the earliest signs of TSC is often the presence of distinct skin findings including hypomelanotic macules (pale patches of skin), facial angiofibromas or bumps over the nose and cheeks, shagreen patches (rough patches of skin), and ungual fibromas (growths under or around the nails). These manifestations are important diagnostic clues and may appear as early as birth.

Central nervous system involvement

Brain involvement is very common in TSC and can lead to a wide range of symptoms, including seizures, intellectual disability, developmental delay, and behavioral problems. In TSC it is common to see benign brain tumors called cortical tubers, subependymal nodules (SENs) and subependymal giant cell astrocytomas (SEGAs). The presence of any of these lesions on brain imaging is highly suggestive of TSC and can aid in diagnosis, even in the absence of overt clinical symptoms.

Visceral involvement

TSC can also affect other organs such as the kidneys, lungs, heart, and eyes. Doctors may look for the presence of renal angiomyolipomas (benign tumors of the kidneys), lymphangioleiomyomatosis (abnormal growth of smooth muscle cells in the lungs), cardiac rhabdomyomas (benign heart tumors), or retinal hamartomas (non-cancerous tumor-like growths on the retina). Diagnosis of TSC in childhood typically involves a combination of clinical assessment and various diagnostic tests. A complete medical history, physical examination, and family history are often the first steps in arriving at a diagnosis. Imaging studies including magnetic resonance imaging (MRI) and computed tomography (CT) scans are also used to identify any central nervous system or visceral involvement. Genetic testing is another important tool for diagnosis, as TSC is an inherited genetic disorder. In conclusion, diagnosing TSC in childhood involves recognizing specific TSC features, performing imaging studies, and genetic testing. Early identification of TSC is important to provide proper treatment and support to children and their families.

CHAPTER 2: DIAGNOSING TUBEROUS SCLEROSIS COMPLEX

Subchapter 2.3: Diagnosis in Adulthood

Although Tuberous Sclerosis Complex (TSC) is typically diagnosed in infants or young children, it is possible for individuals to receive a TSC diagnosis in adulthood. This can happen if a person has only mild symptoms or has not previously sought medical attention for their symptoms. Some common signs and symptoms of TSC that may lead to an adult diagnosis include seizures, kidney problems, skin abnormalities, and cognitive or behavioral issues. If an adult presents with these symptoms, a doctor will typically perform a physical exam and medical history review. In addition, imaging tests such as MRI or CT scans may be conducted to identify any tumors in the brain, kidneys, or other organs. Genetic testing may also be ordered to confirm a TSC diagnosis and determine its severity. It's important for adults who receive a TSC diagnosis to work closely with their healthcare team to develop a treatment plan and manage their symptoms. They should also alert family members to the possibility of inheritance, as TSC is a genetic disorder. Receiving a TSC diagnosis as an adult can feel overwhelming, but with the right support and resources, individuals can still live full and meaningful lives. There are a variety of treatment options available for managing symptoms, and advocacy organizations exist to offer support and connect individuals with others who understand their experiences.

Chapter 3: Treatment Options

Tuberous Sclerosis Complex can manifest itself in a variety of ways, and as such, there are several different types of treatment options available. The primary goal of these treatments is to manage the symptoms of this condition, and to help those diagnosed improve their quality of life.

SUBCHAPTER 3.1: MEDICATIONS

Many medications have been proven effective in treating the symptoms of Tuberous Sclerosis Complex. One of the most commonly used drugs is antiepileptic medication, which is prescribed to manage seizures. Some antiepileptic medications are effective in controlling seizures caused by this condition, and others are prescribed to reduce behavioral symptoms. In addition to antiepileptic medication, there are also medications available to manage skin lesions and tumors caused by Tuberous Sclerosis Complex. These medications are designed to shrink or eliminate the growths to improve cosmetic appearance and reduce discomfort associated with the symptomatic areas.

SUBCHAPTER 3.2: SURGERY

For those with more severe cases of Tuberous Sclerosis Complex, surgery may be an option. Surgery is typically reserved for dealing with large tumors or potentially life-threatening issues, such as a tumor that is obstructing an airway. Surgical intervention can be performed in a number of different ways depending on the patient's specific needs. This includes removing growths or lesions, performing brain surgery to manage epilepsy, or even kidney transplant if symptoms are severe and uncontrollable by medication.

SUBCHAPTER 3.3: THERAPY OPTIONS

Various therapy options exist that can help manage the symptoms of Tuberous Sclerosis Complex. Physical therapy can help maintain motor function and flexibility in those whose movements are impaired by the condition. Occupational therapy can also be useful by teaching those with Tuberous Sclerosis Complex new ways to approach daily tasks that are otherwise becoming difficult for them. There are also psychological therapies available for those affected by the psychological or emotional symptoms that can come along with Tuberous Sclerosis Complex, such as anxiety and depression. Overall, these therapies offer individuals a way to control and manage the symptoms of this condition to live a higher-quality life. It is important to note that individuals may require a combination of treatments, and a personalized approach is recommended to determine the best treatment plan for each individual case. The effectiveness of treatments can vary greatly, and those diagnosed with Tuberous Sclerosis Complex should work closely with their healthcare provider to find the best approach to manage symptoms and improve their overall wellbeing.

SUBCHAPTER 3.1:
MEDICATIONS

Medications can be an effective treatment option for individuals with Tuberous Sclerosis Complex (TSC). However, the type and dosage of medication vary depending on the severity and location of the symptoms. Here are some types of medications commonly used to treat TSC:

Antiepileptic Drugs (AEDs)

AEDs are prescribed to control seizures in people with TSC. There are several options available, such as carbamazepine, lamotrigine, and valproic acid. These medications work by reducing abnormal electrical activity in the brain that causes seizures. It is important to note that AEDs may have side effects, such as drowsiness and dizziness.

Angiotensin-Converting Enzyme (ACE) Inhibitors

ACE inhibitors, such as lisinopril and enalapril, are used to treat kidney tumors and reduce the risk of complications. These medications work by blocking the production of a hormone that causes blood vessels to constrict, which can lead to high blood pressure and kidney damage.

Everolimus

Everolimus is a medication that can shrink or slow the growth of TSC-related tumors. It works by inhibiting a protein that promotes tumor cell growth. This medication is often used to treat kidney and brain tumors in people with TSC. However, everolimus may have side effects, such as mouth sores and infections.

Nicotinamide

Nicotinamide, also known as Vitamin B3, is a medication that has been recently investigated as a potential treatment option for epilepsy in people with TSC. Studies have shown that nicotinamide can reduce seizure frequency and severity, although more research is needed to confirm its effectiveness. Overall, medication is just one of several treatment options available for TSC. It is important to consult with a healthcare professional to determine the best course of treatment for your individual needs.

SUBCHAPTER 3.2: SURGERY

In some cases of tuberous sclerosis complex (TSC), surgery may be necessary to manage the symptoms and complications of the condition. Surgery is typically considered when medication and other non-invasive treatments are not effective. There are several types of surgeries that may be performed for TSC, depending on the individual's specific needs. One common type of surgery is to remove tumors or growths in the body. This may be done through a procedure called a resection, which involves cutting out the affected tissue. In some cases, radiation therapy may also be used to shrink tumors before they are removed surgically. In addition to tumor removal, surgery may also be used to manage seizures in individuals with TSC. One type of surgery that may be performed is called a corpus callosotomy, which involves cutting the corpus callosum (a band of nerve fibers that connects the two halves of the brain) to prevent seizures from spreading between the two hemispheres. Another type of surgery is called a lobectomy, which involves removing a portion of the brain that is generating seizures. It is important to note that surgery for TSC carries risks and potential complications, just like any other type of surgery. However, for some individuals with TSC, surgery can be a valuable treatment option that can greatly improve their quality of life. If you or your loved one with TSC are considering surgery, it is important to speak with your healthcare provider to fully understand the benefits, risks, and potential outcomes. Overall, while surgery is not always necessary for individuals with TSC, it can be an effective treatment option for managing certain symptoms and complications of the condition. If you have any questions or concerns about surgery for TSC, be sure to speak with your doctor or a specialist who is familiar with the condition.

SUBCHAPTER 3.3: THERAPY OPTIONS

In addition to medications and surgery, there are a variety of therapy options available for individuals with Tuberous Sclerosis Complex (TSC). These therapies can help manage symptoms, improve developmental delays and quality of life, and address behavioral and emotional challenges. **Occupational Therapy:** Occupational therapy can help individuals with TSC improve their fine motor skills, coordination, and sensory processing. This can be especially helpful for children with TSC who may struggle with everyday activities such as dressing, eating, and writing. **Physical Therapy:** Physical therapy can help individuals with TSC improve their gross motor skills, balance, and overall physical functioning. This can help individuals maintain or improve their physical abilities. **Speech Therapy:** Speech therapy can help individuals with TSC improve their communication skills. This can include addressing speech and language delays, improving social communication, and addressing feeding and swallowing difficulties. **Behavioral Therapy:** Behavioral therapy can help individuals with TSC manage challenging behaviors and improve social skills. This can include cognitive behavioral therapy (CBT), social skills training, and parent training programs. **Psychological Therapy:** Psychological therapy can help individuals with TSC manage the emotional and psychological challenges that may come with the condition. This can include talk therapy, supportive therapy, and cognitive behavioral therapy (CBT). Overall, therapy options can be an important part of managing TSC symptoms and improving quality of life. It is important to work with a healthcare team to determine which therapies may be most beneficial for each individual with TSC.

Living with Tuberous Sclerosis Complex

Living with Tuberous Sclerosis Complex (TSC) can be challenging, but it's not impossible. Although the symptoms of TSC can vary greatly from person to person, there are some general strategies that can help you manage your symptoms and maintain a good quality of life. In this chapter, we will discuss some of the common challenges faced by people with TSC and provide some tips for managing those challenges.

MANAGING SEIZURES

One of the most common symptoms of TSC is seizures. These can range from mild to severe, and can be a major source of stress for both the person with TSC and their loved ones. If you or someone you know has TSC and experiences seizures, there are several things you can do to help manage them. First and foremost, it's important to work closely with your healthcare provider to find the right medication to control your seizures. Antiepileptic drugs (AEDs) are the most commonly used type of medication for seizures, and there are many different kinds to choose from. Your healthcare provider will work with you to determine which medication is best for you based on your symptoms, medical history, and other factors. In addition to medication, there are some lifestyle changes you can make that may help reduce your risk of seizures. These include getting enough sleep, avoiding alcohol and drugs that can trigger seizures, and reducing stress as much as possible. It can also be helpful to keep a seizure diary to track your symptoms and identify any patterns or triggers that may be contributing to your seizures.

DEALING WITH NEUROLOGICAL ISSUES

In addition to seizures, many people with TSC experience other neurological issues, such as developmental delays, learning disabilities, and behavioral problems. If you or someone you know is dealing with these types of issues, there are several things you can do to help. First, it's important to work closely with your healthcare provider to determine the underlying cause of the issue and identify appropriate treatments. Depending on the specific symptoms, this may include medication, therapy, or other types of interventions. You can also help by providing a supportive and nurturing environment at home. This may involve making adjustments to your home or daily routine to accommodate your loved one's needs, seeking out additional support or resources as needed, and offering plenty of love and encouragement.

MANAGING BEHAVIORAL CHALLENGES

Behavioral issues can be a significant challenge for those with TSC and their loved ones. These may include aggression, impulsivity, and hyperactivity, among other things. If you or someone you know is dealing with these types of issues, it's important to work closely with your healthcare provider to determine appropriate treatments. This may include medication, therapy, or other types of interventions. It can also be helpful to adopt a consistent and structured approach to managing behavior at home. This may involve setting clear rules and expectations, offering rewards for positive behavior, and providing consequences for negative behavior. It's also important to offer plenty of positive reinforcement, such as praise and encouragement, for good behavior.

COPING WITH EMOTIONAL AND PSYCHOLOGICAL EFFECTS

Living with TSC can be emotionally and psychologically challenging, both for the person with TSC and their loved ones. If you or someone you know is struggling with these types of issues, there are several things you can do to help. First, it's important to seek out professional support from a qualified mental health provider. This may include counseling, therapy, or other types of interventions. You can also help by providing emotional support and understanding at home. This may involve listening without judgment, offering reassurance and comfort, and providing opportunities for your loved one to talk about their feelings and concerns.

Conclusion

Living with Tuberous Sclerosis Complex can be challenging, but it's important to remember that you're not alone. By working closely with your healthcare providers, adopting healthy lifestyle practices, and providing a supportive and nurturing environment at home, you can help manage your symptoms and maintain a good quality of life. Remember to take care of yourself, seek out support when needed, and never give up hope.

SUBCHAPTER 4.1: MANAGING SEIZURES

Seizures are a common symptom of Tuberous Sclerosis Complex (TSC), affecting up to 80% of individuals. Seizures can be distressing for both the person experiencing them and their loved ones. Managing seizures can be challenging, but with the right approach, it is possible to reduce their frequency and impact on daily life. The first step in managing seizures in TSC is to work with your doctor to develop a treatment plan. This plan may involve medications to control seizures, such as antiepileptic drugs (AEDs) or anti-seizure medication. It is important to take these medications as prescribed and to let your doctor know if you are experiencing any side effects. Lifestyle modifications can also be helpful in managing seizures. Good sleep habits, reducing stress, and avoiding triggers such as flashing lights or certain foods, can all help to reduce the frequency and severity of seizures. In some cases, surgery or other interventions may be necessary to manage seizures. For example, individuals with TSC who experience seizures that cannot be controlled with medication may be candidates for surgical removal of the part of the brain responsible for the seizures. It is important to keep track of seizures and to communicate any changes or new symptoms to your doctor. Regular check-ins with your doctor can help to adjust your treatment plan as needed and ensure that you are getting the best care possible. Overall, managing seizures in TSC requires a comprehensive approach that includes medical treatment, lifestyle modifications, and ongoing communication with your healthcare provider. With the right approach, it is possible to minimize the impact of seizures on daily life and achieve greater quality of life.

DEALING WITH NEUROLOGICAL ISSUES

Neurological issues are common in individuals with Tuberous Sclerosis Complex (TSC) due to the growth of noncancerous tumors in the brain. These tumors can cause seizures, developmental delays, and intellectual disability, among other problems. It is important to manage these neurological issues to improve the quality of life for those with TSC. One of the primary neurological issues associated with TSC is seizures. Seizures can have a significant impact on daily life and can lead to injury or sudden unexpected death. It is crucial to work with a neurologist who specializes in TSC to develop an individualized treatment plan that may include medications and other therapeutic interventions to manage seizures. In addition to seizures, individuals with TSC may experience developmental delays and intellectual disability, which can impact daily life and limit opportunities. It is important to work with a team of healthcare professionals, including developmental pediatricians, psychologists, and occupational therapists, to address these issues and improve overall functioning. Therapeutic interventions may include speech therapy, occupational therapy, and educational support. Other neurological issues associated with TSC may include autism spectrum disorder, sleep problems, and attention deficit hyperactivity disorder (ADHD). It is important to work with a team of healthcare professionals to identify and manage these issues to improve overall functioning and quality of life. It is important for individuals with TSC and their loved ones to be informed and educated about the neurological issues associated with TSC. By working with a team of healthcare professionals and developing an individualized treatment plan, many of these issues can be managed effectively, and individuals with TSC can live fulfilling lives.# Managing Behavioral Challenges Tuberous Sclerosis Complex (TSC) can cause a wide range of behavioral challenges. These can include hyperactivity, inattention, impulsivity, aggression, anxiety, depression, and self-injury, among others. Managing these challenges can be difficult, but there are strategies that you and your loved ones can use to help manage behavior and reduce the impact it can have on your daily life. Here are some approaches that may help. ## Behavioral Therapy Behavioral therapy can be effective for individuals with TSC. This type of therapy focuses on altering behaviors that are disruptive or harmful, developing healthy coping mechanisms, and improving social and communication skills. There are many different types of behavioral therapy, including cognitive behavioral therapy (CBT), dialectical behavioral therapy (DBT), and applied behavior analysis (ABA). A trained therapist can work with you or your loved one to identify problematic behaviors and develop strategies to improve them. This may include setting goals, developing coping strategies, practicing problem-solving skills, and using positive reinforcement to encourage positive behaviors. ## Medications In some cases, medication may be prescribed to help manage behavioral challenges associated with TSC. Anticonvulsant medications may be used to help control seizures, which can sometimes improve behavior as well. Other medications, such as antidepressants or mood stabilizers, may be used to help manage anxiety, depression, and other mood disorders. It is important to work closely with your healthcare provider when taking medications and to monitor for side effects that may impact behavior. ##

Lifestyle Modifications Lifestyle modifications can also be helpful in managing behavioral challenges associated with TSC. This may include establishing a consistent daily routine, getting enough sleep, eating a healthy diet, and implementing relaxation techniques like deep breathing and meditation. Exercise can also be beneficial for managing behavior, as it can help reduce stress and promote the release of endorphins, which can improve mood. Activities like yoga, swimming, and cycling may be particularly helpful. ## Creating a Supportive Environment Creating a supportive environment can also be critical in managing behavioral challenges associated with TSC. This may involve setting clear boundaries and expectations, using positive reinforcement to encourage positive behaviors, and providing a safe and structured environment for your loved one. It is also important to provide opportunities for social interaction and support, as social isolation can contribute to behavioral challenges.

Managing the behavioral challenges associated with TSC can be challenging, but these strategies can be effective in promoting positive behaviors and improving quality of life. By working closely with your healthcare provider and implementing these approaches, you can help reduce the impact that TSC has on your daily life.

SUBCHAPTER 4.4: COPING WITH EMOTIONAL AND PSYCHOLOGICAL EFFECTS

Dealing with Tuberous Sclerosis Complex (TSC) can be mentally and emotionally exhausting not only for the patient but also their loved ones. Coping with emotional and psychological effects can be a huge challenge, but with the right tools and support, it can be managed. It is common for individuals with TSC to experience anxiety, depression, and behavioral challenges. These challenges arise due to the physical symptoms of TSC or simply the stress associated with having a chronic condition. It is important to consult with a mental health professional to manage these challenges effectively. Behavioral challenges such as aggression, impulsivity, and hyperactivity are common among individuals with TSC. Developing strategies to handle these behaviors can help individuals and caregivers manage them better. One effective strategy is behavior modification which includes positive reinforcement and consistency in discipline. It is essential to create a supportive environment for individuals with TSC. Having a support team that consists of family members, doctors, therapists, and community resources can positively impact an individual's mental health. It is also essential to note that caregivers need support too. The stress of caring for a loved one with TSC can take a toll on their mental and emotional health. Caregivers must take care of their own emotional and mental health. In conclusion, coping with the emotional and psychological effects of TSC can be challenging, but with the right support, it can be managed. Getting the appropriate mental health support, developing effective strategies to manage behavioral challenges, and creating a supportive environment can help individuals with TSC and their loved ones to cope better.

Chapter 5: Tuberous Sclerosis Complex and Your Children

If you have a child who has been diagnosed with tuberous sclerosis complex (TSC), it's completely natural to feel overwhelmed and uncertain about what the future holds. However, with the right support and resources, you and your child can navigate life with TSC and thrive. In this chapter, we will cover some tips and strategies for supporting your child with TSC, from diagnosis to adulthood.

SUBCHAPTER 5.1:
ADVOCATING FOR YOUR CHILD

As a parent, one of the most important roles you play is that of an advocate for your child. This is especially true when your child has a chronic condition like TSC. Here are some tips for effective advocacy:

1. Educate Yourself

The more you know about TSC, the better equipped you will be to advocate for your child. Research the condition, its symptoms, and treatment options. Attend local TSC support groups and conferences to connect with other families and learn from their experiences.

2. Build a Strong Support Network

Surround yourself and your child with a team of healthcare professionals who are knowledgeable about TSC. This may include a neurologist, a geneticist, a psychiatrist, and a developmental pediatrician. You may also want to work with a case manager who can help you navigate the healthcare system and connect you with community resources.

3. Communicate Effectively

When advocating for your child, it's important to communicate clearly and effectively with healthcare providers, educators, and other members of your child's support team. Keep detailed records of your child's symptoms, medications, and treatments. Share this information with your child's healthcare team and be proactive about asking questions and expressing concerns.

SUBCHAPTER 5.2: MANAGING THE DIAGNOSIS

Receiving a diagnosis of TSC can be a scary and overwhelming experience for both you and your child. Here are some tips for managing the diagnosis:

1. Be Honest

It's important to be honest with your child about their diagnosis, in an age-appropriate way. Use simple and clear language to explain the condition, and emphasize that it's not their fault. Reassure your child that they are not alone, and that you will be there to support them every step of the way.

2. Address Any Behavioral Challenges

Children with TSC may experience behavioral challenges such as aggression, impulsivity, and hyperactivity. It's important to address these challenges early on with a healthcare professional who is knowledgeable about TSC. They may recommend behavioral therapy, medication, or other interventions to help your child manage their symptoms.

3. Advocate for Your Child's Education

Children with TSC may need accommodations in the classroom to help them succeed academically. Work with your child's teachers and school administrators to develop an individualized education plan (IEP) that outlines your child's specific needs and accommodations. Be persistent in advocating for your child's needs, and don't hesitate to seek outside help if necessary.

SUBCHAPTER 5.3: SUPPORTING YOUR CHILD'S EMOTIONAL NEEDS

Children with TSC may experience a wide range of emotions, from fear and anxiety to frustration and anger. As a parent, it's important to support your child's emotional needs. Here are some tips:

1. Encourage Open Communication

Encourage your child to talk about their feelings, and listen actively without judgment. If your child is having trouble expressing themselves verbally, encourage them to draw or write in a journal.

2. Provide a Safe and Supportive Home Environment

Create a home environment that is safe, supportive, and predictable. Stick to regular routines and schedules, and minimize changes or disruptions as much as possible. Provide your child with plenty of love, affection, and positive reinforcement.

3. Connect with Other Families

Connecting with other families who are in similar situations can be a valuable source of support for both you and your child. Attend local TSC support groups or connect with other families online through social media or online forums. Remember, you and your child are not alone in navigating life with TSC. With the right support and resources, your family can thrive and achieve a high quality of life.

CHAPTER 5: TUBEROUS SCLEROSIS COMPLEX AND YOUR CHILDREN

Subchapter 5.1: Advocating for Your Child

If your child has been diagnosed with Tuberous Sclerosis Complex (TSC), it is important as a parent to become an advocate for their health and wellbeing. This means learning as much as possible about the condition, and communicating with healthcare providers and educators on behalf of your child. One important step in advocating for your child is ensuring they receive proper medical care. This may involve coordinating care between multiple healthcare providers, monitoring medication side effects, and keeping track of appointments and medical records. It is also important to communicate effectively with your child's educators, particularly if they have special needs due to TSC. This may involve creating an individualized education plan with the school, ensuring accommodations are in place to support your child's learning, and advocating for appropriate classroom placements and resources. Additionally, advocating for your child with TSC may involve raising awareness of the condition in your community, advocating for increased research funding, and supporting organizations that provide resources and services for individuals and families affected by TSC. Remember, you are your child's greatest advocate. By staying informed, communicating effectively, and advocating for their needs, you can help your child with TSC lead a fulfilling and successful life.

MANAGING THE DIAGNOSIS

Receiving a diagnosis of Tuberous Sclerosis Complex can be overwhelming for both parents and children alike. Once you have received a diagnosis, it's important to take certain steps to manage and cope with the condition. Firstly, it's essential to develop a good working relationship with your healthcare provider. They can provide you with essential information and support throughout the diagnosis and treatment process. They can also guide you in managing your child's symptoms and offer resources for additional support. After receiving a diagnosis, make sure you ask your healthcare provider as many questions as you need. Make a list of questions before each visit, so you don't forget them. Ask about immediate treatment options and long-term management strategies. Once you have more information about TSC, it's important to inform your child's school, caregiver, and close friends and family about the diagnosis. Educate them about the condition and how it affects your child. This will help build a support system for your child and reduce the risk of bullying or exclusion. Finally, be proactive in monitoring your child's health. Keep track of their symptoms and keep a record of any new developments. Report any changes to your healthcare provider immediately. This will help you stay ahead of any potential complications and maintain your child's overall health and wellbeing. Remember, managing your child's TSC diagnosis is a team effort. Stay informed, communicate with your healthcare provider and support system, and stay proactive in monitoring your child's health. This will help you provide the best care and support for your child.

CHAPTER 5: TUBEROUS SCLEROSIS COMPLEX AND YOUR CHILDREN

Subchapter 5.3: Supporting Your Child's Emotional Needs

Children with Tuberous Sclerosis Complex (TSC) not only deal with physical challenges but also emotional and psychological ones. The diagnosis can be overwhelming for both the child and their family, so it's important to support your child's emotional and mental well-being. One of the main emotional needs your child may have is a sense of normalcy. It's important to allow your child to participate in regular activities such as school, sports, and social events. Encourage your child to pursue their interests and hobbies, even if they need some modifications to participate. It's also important to communicate with your child regularly and create a safe environment where they feel comfortable expressing their emotions. Understand that your child may feel frustrated or discouraged at times, and it's important to validate their feelings and offer support. Seeking out a licensed therapist or counselor can also be beneficial for both your child and your family. Therapists can provide coping mechanisms and emotional support to help your child navigate their feelings and challenges related to their TSC diagnosis. Lastly, providing resources and support groups for your child can create a sense of community and belonging. Your child may benefit from meeting others with TSC and realizing they are not alone in their struggles. By supporting your child's emotional needs, you can help them lead a fulfilling life and cope with the challenges that come with TSC.

Chapter 6: Navigating Life with Tuberous Sclerosis Complex

Living with Tuberous Sclerosis Complex (TSC) can be a challenging experience, but the right support and resources can make all the difference. In this chapter, we will discuss various ways to navigate life with TSC and to help you overcome some of the challenges that you may face.

SUBCHAPTER 6.1: BUILDING A SUPPORT TEAM

One of the most important things that you can do when living with TSC is to build a strong support team. This team should consist of medical professionals, family members, and friends who can provide emotional support and practical assistance. Your medical team should be knowledgeable about TSC and should include specialists who can help address the various aspects of the condition, such as neurologists, dermatologists, and psychiatrists. These professionals can work together to create a comprehensive care plan tailored to your individual needs. In addition to medical professionals, it is important to have a support system of family and friends. This can help you deal with the challenges of TSC and help you maintain a positive outlook.

SUBCHAPTER 6.2: MAKING LIFESTYLE ADJUSTMENTS

Living with TSC often requires making adjustments to your lifestyle. This may include changes to your diet, exercise routine, and daily activities. For example, some people with TSC may need to avoid certain foods or substances that can trigger seizures or other symptoms. Others may need to modify their exercise routine to reduce the risk of injury. Making these adjustments can be challenging, but it is important to remember that they can help you manage your symptoms and live a healthier life.

SUBCHAPTER 6.3: ADVOCATING FOR YOURSELF

Advocating for yourself is an important part of navigating life with TSC. This means speaking up for your needs and rights and being proactive in seeking out resources and support. There are many resources available to help individuals with TSC and their families. These include support groups, educational materials, and advocacy organizations. By staying informed and involved in your care, you can take an active role in managing your TSC and ensuring that you receive the best possible treatment and support. In conclusion, navigating life with TSC can be challenging, but with the right support and resources, it is possible to live a full and rewarding life. By building a strong support team, making necessary lifestyle adjustments, and advocating for yourself, you can manage your symptoms and overcome the challenges of TSC.

BUILDING A SUPPORT TEAM

Building a support team is crucial when navigating life with Tuberous Sclerosis Complex (TSC). This team may consist of healthcare professionals, family members, friends, and support groups. It is important to have people who understand your unique situation and can support you both emotionally and physically. One of the most essential members of your support team will be your healthcare provider. It is important to find a healthcare provider who has experience and knowledge about TSC. They can help you manage your symptoms and provide guidance on treatment options. Family members and friends can also be great sources of support. They can help you with daily tasks, provide emotional support, and offer a listening ear when you need it. It is important to educate them about TSC so they can better understand your needs and how to support you. Support groups are also a valuable resource for individuals and families affected by TSC. These groups provide a sense of community, a safe space to share experiences, and an opportunity to connect with other people who understand what you are going through. Consider joining a support group in your area or online to connect with others who can relate to your experiences. In addition to these key support team members, there may be other healthcare professionals such as therapists or social workers who can provide additional support. They can offer resources and strategies to help manage the emotional and psychological effects of TSC. Remember that building a support team takes time and effort, but it is an important step in navigating life with TSC. Don't be afraid to reach out for help and know that you are not alone in this journey.

SUBCHAPTER 6.2: MAKING LIFESTYLE ADJUSTMENTS

Tuberous Sclerosis Complex requires significant adaptations to daily living. Adjusting to a new lifestyle and managing the effects of TSC can be a difficult and overwhelming experience for both individuals with TSC and their families. It is essential to learn new ways to cope and focus on improving your quality of life. One of the most critical aspects of making lifestyle adjustments is creating a daily routine. Having a structured routine can help reduce stress and anxiety by making daily tasks more manageable. Schedule activities such as taking medications, attending appointments, therapy sessions, and daily exercises at the same time every day. A balanced and nutritious diet is also vital to managing the symptoms of TSC.

Proper nutrition can help ensure a healthy weight and reduce the risk of certain complications. Talk with a professional dietician to create a personalized diet plan that meets specific dietary needs. Individuals with TSC may need to make modifications to their home environment, depending on their condition's severity. Taking care of home maintenance, ensuring safety, removing tripping hazards, and installing supportive tools such as handrails, ramps, shower grab-bars, and toilet risers, can be beneficial. Regular exercise can help improve overall health and maintain mobility, strength, and flexibility. Work with your healthcare provider to develop an exercise program that is safe and appropriate for your condition. Vocational rehabilitation services, career counseling, and job coaching may be necessary for individuals with TSC. These services can assist with developing job skills, finding employment opportunities, and creating a supportive work environment. Making lifestyle adjustments can be a daunting task, but with the right knowledge, support, and resources, individuals with TSC can improve their quality of life and manage their condition effectively.

ADVOCATING FOR YOURSELF

Living with Tuberous Sclerosis Complex is an ongoing challenge that requires you to advocate for yourself. It is essential to be well-informed about your condition and understand your rights. Having a clear understanding of your rights is crucial when it comes to accessing healthcare and receiving appropriate treatment. As an individual with Tuberous Sclerosis Complex, you have the right to speak up and express your needs. It is important to communicate effectively with your healthcare providers to ensure that you receive the best possible care. If you have concerns or questions about your treatments, medication, or any aspect of your care, do not hesitate to ask your healthcare provider. You also have the right to educate yourself about your condition and the available treatments. This means reading medical literature and staying informed about any new studies or therapies that may be available. By educating yourself, you can become a more active participant in your care and feel empowered with the knowledge to advocate for yourself. Finally, you have the right to seek additional resources and support beyond your healthcare providers. Joining support groups or online communities can provide you with a valuable network of individuals who share similar experiences and can offer emotional support, advice, and insights into managing life with Tuberous Sclerosis Complex. In conclusion, advocating for yourself requires taking ownership of your medical care and speaking up about your needs. By educating yourself, communicating effectively with your healthcare providers, and seeking out additional resources and support, you can become a powerful advocate for yourself and live a full and meaningful life with Tuberous Sclerosis Complex.

Chapter 7: Research and Progress

Tuberous Sclerosis Complex (TSC) is a rare genetic disorder, and extensive research is being conducted to better understand it. The development of new treatments is essential, and scientists around the world are working towards finding one. This chapter will provide an overview of the latest research and ongoing clinical trials.

SUBCHAPTER 7.1: OVERVIEW OF THE LATEST RESEARCH

In recent years, there has been significant progress in the research for TSC. Scientists and medical professionals are working together to identify new targeted treatments that can significantly improve the quality of life for people with TSC. One major area of study is the genetic basis of TSC.

Researchers are using cutting-edge genomic technologies to study the genes involved in TSC. The hope is to identify new targets for treatment and gain a deeper understanding of the disorder. Additionally, researchers are investigating the link between epilepsy and TSC. This is because seizures are common in people with TSC, and developing better treatments for them is critical. By understanding the mechanisms of TSC-related seizures, researchers may be able to develop more effective treatments. Another area of research is investigating the role of mTOR signaling in TSC. mTOR is a protein kinase that plays a critical role in a variety of cellular processes, including cell growth and division. It has been linked to TSC and is a focus of ongoing research.

SUBCHAPTER 7.2: CLINICAL TRIALS AND NEW TREATMENTS

Clinical trials represent a critical part of the process for developing new treatments for

TSC. These trials help to ensure that new therapies are safe and effective before they are offered to the public. Many clinical trials are currently underway, and several shows a great deal of promise. One clinical trial has been studying the use of Simvastatin as a treatment for TSC. Simvastatin is a cholesterol-lowering drug that has also been shown to reduce the size of TSC-related brain tumors. This drug has shown promise in the treatment of TSC and is currently undergoing further clinical trials. Another clinical trial has been testing the efficacy of everolimus in treating TSC. Everolimus is an mTOR inhibitor that has been used in cancer treatment. It has also shown promise in treating TSC-related seizures and facial angiofibromas. In addition to these ongoing clinical trials, researchers are developing new treatments for TSC. Many of these treatments target specific cellular pathways that are affected by the disorder.

Conclusion

The ongoing research in the field of TSC is incredibly promising. Advances in genomic technologies, physician collaboration, and clinical trials continue to contribute to the development of new treatments. Additionally, as medical professionals gain a deeper understanding of the underlying mechanisms of TSC, they will be able to provide more targeted treatments that can improve the quality of life for people with this disorder.

SUBCHAPTER 7.1: OVERVIEW OF THE LATEST RESEARCH

Tuberous sclerosis complex (TSC) is a rare genetic disorder that affects various organ systems throughout the body. There has been ongoing research to deepen our understanding of the biology and progression of TSC, as well as to find novel treatments for this disorder. In this subchapter, we will provide an overview of the latest research on TSC. Recent studies have improved our knowledge of the underlying genetic causes of TSC, which has opened up new therapeutic targets. One of the most notable breakthroughs has been the identification of the TSC1 and TSC2 genes, which are responsible for regulating cell growth and proliferation. Mutations in these genes lead to over-activation of the mTOR pathway, which is responsible for the formation of benign tumors in TSC patients. Researchers are currently investigating ways to target the mTOR pathway to reduce tumor growth in TSC patients. Another area of research focuses on improving our understanding of the neurological symptoms of TSC, such as seizures and cognitive deficits. Recent studies have identified many potential mechanisms, including alterations in synaptic function, neuronal migration, and dendritic spine formation. Targeting these mechanisms with new therapies could help to reduce the neurological symptoms of TSC and improve the quality of life for affected individuals. Research is also ongoing to identify biomarkers that can help to diagnose and monitor TSC. Biomarkers are measurable substances or indicators that can be used to track disease progression and response to treatment. Recent studies have identified potential biomarkers, such as the level of certain proteins in the blood or cerebrospinal fluid. The use of biomarkers could lead to earlier diagnosis and more personalized treatment plans for individuals with TSC. Overall, the latest research on TSC is promising and offers hope for improved treatment options and outcomes for individuals with this disorder. However, there is still much to be learned about TSC, and continued research is essential to advance our understanding of this complex disorder.

SUBCHAPTER 7.2: CLINICAL TRIALS AND NEW TREATMENTS

Clinical trials offer a way to test new treatments and therapies before they become available to the public. These trials are tightly regulated to ensure that new treatments are safe and effective. For individuals with Tuberous Sclerosis Complex, clinical trials offer the potential for new and improved treatments that can help manage symptoms and improve overall quality of life. Recent trials have focused on a variety of potential treatments, from medications to surgical interventions. One potential treatment that may be of interest to individuals with TSC is rapamycin, which has been shown to reduce tumor growth in individuals with TSC. Other trials have explored the use of gene therapy as a way to target the underlying genetic causes of TSC. Participating in a clinical trial can be a way to access new treatments that may not yet be available to the public. However, it's important to talk to your doctor and carefully consider the risks and benefits before making a decision to participate.

How to Find Clinical Trials

Clinical trials are typically located at research centers and hospitals throughout the country. The best way to find trials that are currently recruiting participants is to search online registries, such as ClinicalTrials.gov. Your doctor may also be able to provide recommendations and help you determine whether a clinical trial is a good option for you. It's important to carefully consider the potential risks and benefits before enrolling in any clinical trial.

The Future of Tuberous Sclerosis Complex Treatment

As new research emerges on the causes and treatment of TSC, the outlook for individuals with this condition continues to improve. Clinical trials and other research studies offer opportunities to improve our understanding of TSC and develop new and more effective treatment options. Advocacy groups and individuals can play an important role in raising awareness of TSC and supporting research efforts. Through participation in advocacy efforts and research studies, individuals with TSC and their families can help ensure that new treatment options continue to be developed and refined. In the coming years, it's likely that new treatments and therapies will become available to individuals with TSC. However, it's important to continue to raise awareness of TSC and advocate for increased research funding to help ensure that progress continues to be made. Overall, while there is still much to learn about Tuberous Sclerosis Complex, there is reason for hope. Through increased awareness, research, and advocacy efforts, individuals with TSC and their families can help improve treatment options and ultimately improve quality of life for those living with this condition.

Chapter 8: Moving Forward

Moving forward with a diagnosis of Tuberous Sclerosis Complex (TSC) may seem daunting, but it is important to remember that there is hope and support for individuals and families. In this chapter, we will discuss the importance of advocacy and finding hope and support.

SUBCHAPTER 8.1: THE IMPORTANCE OF ADVOCACY

Advocacy is crucial for individuals and families affected by TSC. This can mean advocating for yourself or a loved one when it comes to treatment options, medical care, and education. It is important to understand your rights and the resources available to you. One way to advocate for yourself or your loved one is to connect with national and local TSC organizations. These organizations can provide information and support, as well as advocate on behalf of individuals and families affected by TSC. Another way to advocate is to participate in clinical trials and research studies. This can help to advance the understanding of TSC and lead to new treatments and therapies. Advocacy can also mean speaking out about TSC and raising awareness. This can be done through sharing personal stories, participating in fundraising events, and educating others about the condition.

SUBCHAPTER 8.2: FINDING HOPE AND SUPPORT

Finding hope and support is essential for individuals and families affected by TSC. This can come in many forms, from connecting with others who understand the challenges of TSC to finding new treatments and therapies. One way to find hope and support is to join TSC support groups and online communities. These communities can provide a safe space to connect with others, share information and experiences, and gain emotional support. It is also important to seek out medical professionals who are knowledgeable about TSC and can provide specialized care and treatment options. Participating in research studies and clinical trials can also provide hope for the future of TSC treatment and management. Above all, remember that you are not alone. There is a strong community of individuals and families affected by TSC, and together we can find hope and support for a brighter tomorrow.

CONCLUSION

Moving forward with a TSC diagnosis can be challenging, but there are resources available to help individuals and families navigate the journey. Advocacy, finding hope and support, and participating in research are all crucial components of managing TSC and finding new treatments and therapies. Remember that you are not alone, and there is a community of support available to you.

SUBCHAPTER 8.1: THE IMPORTANCE OF ADVOCACY

Advocacy is a crucial aspect of living with tuberous sclerosis complex (TSC). It involves standing up for your rights and those of your loved ones, and working to ensure that you have access to the resources and support you need to manage this condition. One of the most significant benefits of advocacy is that it can help you feel empowered and in control of your life. When you advocate for yourself or your child with TSC, you may feel more confident and capable. You may also develop new skills and strengths as you learn how to navigate the healthcare system, communicate with doctors and other professionals, and manage the challenges of this condition. Advocacy can also have a positive impact on the broader TSC community. By speaking out about the needs and experiences of people with this condition, you can help to raise awareness, generate support, and create positive change. When you come together with other advocates, you can work to change policies, raise funds for research, and advocate for the needs of your community. There are many different ways to get involved in advocacy for TSC. Some people participate in local support groups or online communities, while others may become involved in advocacy organizations, such as the Tuberous Sclerosis Alliance. You can also get involved by sharing your story with others, writing to your elected representatives, or volunteering your time or resources to TSC-related causes. Whatever form your advocacy takes, it is important to remember that your voice matters. By speaking up and working to create change, you can help to improve life for people with TSC and their families. You can also make a difference in the lives of future generations, by advocating for research that can lead to new treatments and eventually a cure for this condition. In the next subchapter, we will explore different ways to find hope and support as you navigate life with TSC.

SUBCHAPTER 8.2: FINDING HOPE AND SUPPORT

Living with Tuberous Sclerosis Complex (TSC) can be overwhelming and challenging, and it is normal to feel anxious, sad, or even hopeless at times. However, it is crucial to remember that you are not alone, and there is hope and help available. Seeking out support and resources can improve your quality of life and give you the strength to face the challenges of TSC. One excellent resource for people with TSC and their families is the Tuberous Sclerosis Alliance (TS Alliance). The TS Alliance is a national nonprofit organization dedicated to finding a cure for TSC while improving the lives of those affected by it. The organization provides a wealth of information and resources, including educational programs, support groups, and advocacy efforts. Their website also offers a comprehensive list of TSC clinics and providers, as well as a directory of specialists and research studies. Another excellent resource is the Tuberous Sclerosis Complex Global Registry. This online platform is designed to collect and analyze data about people with TSC, with the goal of improving diagnosis, treatment, and overall care. By joining the registry, you can contribute to the advancement of TSC research and connect with other people in the TSC community. Support groups can also be a valuable source of comfort and guidance for people with TSC. There are many online and in-person support groups available, including those run by the TS Alliance, TSC Clinic Network, and other organizations. Connecting with people who share similar experiences can provide you with a sense of community and reduce feelings of isolation. You may also find it helpful to seek therapy or counseling to manage the emotional impact of TSC. A mental health professional can help you develop coping strategies, enhance your resilience, and improve your overall mental wellbeing. They can also provide support to other family members who may be affected by TSC. In conclusion, finding hope and support is crucial for people with TSC and their families. By accessing available resources, joining support groups, and seeking out professional help, you can improve your quality of life and learn to manage the challenges of TSC. Remember that you are not alone, and there is a community of people dedicated to supporting and empowering you.

Resources for Individuals and Families

Living with Tuberous Sclerosis Complex (TSC) can be challenging both physically and emotionally for individuals and their families. Fortunately, there are many resources available to help those affected by the disorder. In this chapter, we will explore some of the best resources and organizations that provide support for TSC.

SUBCHAPTER 9.1: NATIONAL AND LOCAL ORGANIZATIONS

There are many organizations that offer support, education, and advocacy for individuals and families living with TSC. The Tuberous Sclerosis Alliance (TS Alliance) is one of the most prominent national organizations dedicated to supporting individuals with TSC and their families. They offer a variety of resources including informational materials, support groups, and a helpline staffed by trained professionals. The TS Alliance also sponsors research and advocates for policies that benefit individuals with TSC. There are also many local organizations that provide support groups and resources for families affected by TSC. Local organizations can help connect families with resources and support that are specific to their community. Some larger cities may have their own TSC clinics, which can provide specialized medical care and support for individuals with TSC and their families. To find local organizations and clinics, the TS Alliance website is a great resource.

SUBCHAPTER 9.2: ONLINE COMMUNITIES

The Internet has made it easier for individuals and families affected by TSC to connect with one another and share information. There are many online communities dedicated to TSC where individuals and families can find support, share stories, and ask questions. Some of the most popular online communities include Facebook groups and online forums. The TS Alliance offers an online community for individuals and families affected by TSC. The community is a safe and supportive space for sharing experiences and asking questions. The TS Alliance community is moderated to ensure that it remains a positive and helpful resource for all members.

SUBCHAPTER 9.3: ADDITIONAL RESOURCES AND SUPPORT

In addition to the resources mentioned above, there are many other resources available to support individuals and families affected by TSC. The National Institutes of Health (NIH) provides up-to-date information on TSC research and treatment options. Other organizations, such as the Tuberous Sclerosis Complex International (TSCi), offer support and resources for families worldwide. There are also many books and publications available on TSC, including medical texts, memoirs, and informational resources. Ask your healthcare provider or local library for recommendations.

The Bottom Line

Living with TSC can be difficult, but it is important to know that there are many resources available to help individuals and families affected by this disorder. From national organizations to local support groups, from online forums to published materials, there is support out there for those who need it. Don't be afraid to reach out for help or to connect with others who share similar experiences.

SUBCHAPTER 9.1: NATIONAL AND LOCAL ORGANIZATIONS

Living with Tuberous Sclerosis Complex can be difficult, but thankfully there are resources available to help individuals and families navigate this condition. National and local organizations can provide access to valuable information, support, and resources. One such organization is the Tuberous Sclerosis Alliance (TS Alliance), a non-profit organization dedicated to finding a cure for Tuberous Sclerosis Complex while improving the lives of those affected by it. The TS Alliance offers a wide range of support services, including educational resources, advocacy, and research. They also have a comprehensive database of clinical trials for TSC. Other national organizations include the National Organization for Rare Disorders (NORD) and the Genetic and Rare Diseases Information Center (GARD). These organizations provide a variety of resources and support to individuals and families living with rare diseases, including TSC. In addition to national organizations, there are also numerous local organizations that provide support and resources for individuals and families affected by TSC. These organizations may include local chapters of national organizations or independent non-profits. If you are looking for local resources, a good place to start is by contacting your local hospital or medical center. They may be able to provide you with information about local support groups or organizations. Overall, there are many national and local organizations that can provide support and resources for individuals and families affected by TSC. Don't hesitate to reach out and connect with these organizations for assistance in navigating this complex condition. Next, we will discuss online communities for TSC support.

One in a Million: Navigating Life with Tuberous Sclerosis Complex

SUBCHAPTER 9.2: ONLINE COMMUNITIES

Living with Tuberous Sclerosis Complex can be challenging, but having a support system can make a difference. While family and friends can provide emotional support, connecting with others who share similar experiences can be valuable. In today's digital age, online communities have become an increasingly popular way for individuals to connect with others who are also managing Tuberous Sclerosis Complex. There are several online communities dedicated to Tuberous Sclerosis Complex where individuals and families can find support and information. These communities are usually run by organizations or are forums created by individuals and can be found with a simple internet search. One such community is the Tuberous Sclerosis Alliance (TS Alliance). TS Alliance is a nonprofit organization dedicated to finding a cure for TSC and improving the lives of those affected. They offer an online community forum where individuals and families can connect with one another, share their experiences, and support each other. Another community is the Tuberous Sclerosis Complex Support Group on Facebook. This group was created by individuals affected by TSC and has grown to over 6,000 members. It provides support, information, and a safe space for individuals to share their experiences. The Tuberous Sclerosis Complex Forum on RareConnect is another online community that provides a safe and supportive environment for individuals and families affected by TSC. The forum is moderated and provides access to medical professionals and experts who can answer questions and provide guidance. Online communities can be a great resource for individuals and families affected by Tuberous Sclerosis Complex. They can provide emotional support, information, resources, and a sense of community. However, it is important to remember that online communities should not replace medical advice and guidance from healthcare professionals. In conclusion, if you or someone you know is affected by Tuberous Sclerosis Complex, consider joining an online community. It can provide a sense of belonging and a valuable support system.

SUBCHAPTER 9.3: ADDITIONAL RESOURCES AND SUPPORT

In addition to national and local organizations and online communities, there are many other resources available for individuals and families affected by Tuberous Sclerosis Complex. One great resource is the Tuberous Sclerosis Alliance, which offers a wide variety of information and support for individuals and families, including resources for education, advocacy, and research. They also offer a referral service to help individuals find doctors and medical facilities that specialize in the treatment of Tuberous Sclerosis Complex. Another valuable resource is the Tuberous Sclerosis Complex Clinic Network, which brings together doctors and specialists from around the country to provide comprehensive care for individuals with Tuberous Sclerosis Complex. Through this network, individuals and families can access the latest treatments and therapies, as well as participate in research studies and clinical trials. Lastly, there are many support groups available for individuals and families affected by Tuberous Sclerosis Complex. These groups can provide a safe and supportive environment for individuals to discuss their experiences, share information, and connect with others who understand what they are going through. Many of these groups are available both online and in person, and can be a great source of comfort and encouragement. No matter what stage of the journey you are on, it's important to remember that you are not alone. There are many resources and support available for individuals and families affected by Tuberous Sclerosis Complex, and with the right information and support, you can navigate the challenges and find hope for the future.

Conclusion

In conclusion, Tuberous Sclerosis Complex (TSC) is a rare genetic disorder that affects multiple parts of the body, including the brain, skin, kidneys, heart, lungs, and eyes. There is no cure for the condition, but treatments are available to manage symptoms and improve quality of life. Throughout this book, we have discussed the various aspects of TSC, from understanding the signs and symptoms to diagnosis, treatment options, and coping with the condition. We have also explored the impact of TSC on children and families and discussed how to navigate life with this complex disorder. It is important to note that TSC is not a one-size-fits-all condition. Each person with TSC is different and may experience different symptoms and challenges. However, with proper diagnosis, treatment, and support, individuals with TSC can lead fulfilling and rewarding lives. Advocacy and research continue to be crucial in the fight against TSC, and new treatments are currently in development. It is important for individuals with TSC and their families to stay informed about the latest developments and to be active participants in their own care.

Finally, it is essential to acknowledge the strength and resilience of those living with TSC. Managing a chronic condition can be challenging both physically and emotionally, but with the right mindset and support, anything is possible. Thank you for reading One in a Million: Navigating Life with Tuberous Sclerosis Complex. We hope this book has provided you with valuable information and insight into this complex condition. Remember, you are not alone in this journey, and together, we can continue to raise awareness and find new ways to support those living with TSC.

About the Author

As the author of "One in a Million: Navigating Life with Tuberous Sclerosis Complex," I have a personal connection to this topic. I am a parent of a child who has been diagnosed with TSC, and I have also been an advocate for individuals and families affected by this condition for many years. Through my journey, I have learned how challenging it can be to navigate life with TSC. However, I have also learned that with the right support and resources, it is possible to live a fulfilling life despite the challenges. Writing this book has been a passion project for me, and I am grateful for the opportunity to share my knowledge and experience with others. My hope is that this book will serve as a helpful guide for individuals and families who are navigating life with TSC, and that it will provide valuable insight and resources for anyone who is interested in learning more about this condition. Thank you for taking the time to read "One in a Million: Navigating Life with Tuberous Sclerosis Complex." I hope that it will be informative, empowering, and inspiring for you.